# EMBRACING A RAW FOOD LIFESTYLE

## The Raw Food Revolution

JENNIFER M.LUX

# TABLE OF CONTENTS

# INTRODUCTION

## An introduction to adopting a raw food lifestyle

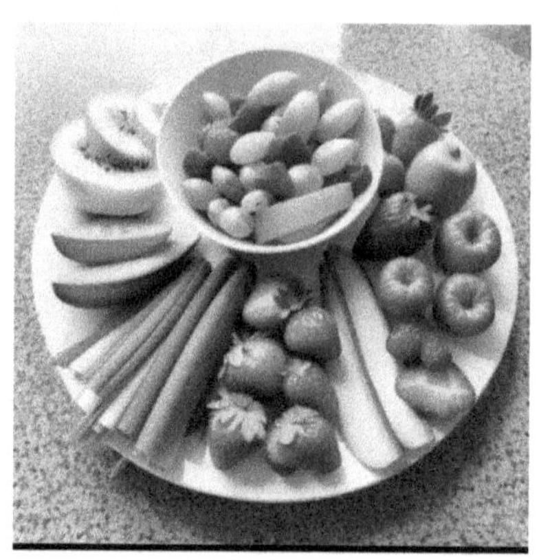

Paulina's journey towards better health began when she stumbled upon a book called "EMBRACING A RAW FOOD LIFESTYLE" by Jennifer M. Lux.

It was a turning point in her life that set her on the path of renewal and transformation.

The book fully explained the benefits of adopting a raw food lifestyle, highlighting the potential for healing, restoring, and alleviating various health conditions.

Paulina, interested and determined to improve her health, decided to give it a try. For many years, Paulina suffered from a chronic autoimmune disease that left her with frequent fatigue, joint pain, and infections.

She has tried many traditional remedies and medicines, but none of them brought her the relief she was looking for.

Frustrated by the limitations of conventional medicine, she turned to alternative methods and eventually discovered the raw food lifestyle.

Jennifer M. Lux's book provides an in-depth understanding of the raw food diet, describing the principles, benefits, and success stories of individuals who have undergone remarkable transformations.

Paulina is fascinated by the testimonials of people who have improved their health by eating fresh foods.

The book explains that a raw food lifestyle primarily includes the consumption of fresh, uncooked fruits, vegetables, nuts, and seeds.

She stresses the importance of avoiding processed and cooked foods, as they can lose essential nutrients during the cooking process.

The author points out that raw foods are rich in enzymes, vitamins, minerals, and antioxidants, which can promote healing and detoxification in the body.

Eager to apply these principles to her daily life, Paulina embarked on a journey of discovery. She began incorporating more raw fruits and vegetables into her diet, and gradually eliminating processed foods and cooked foods from her meals.

The transition was difficult at first because she was used to ready-to-eat foods. Still, she persisted, motivated by the potential benefits she could reap from it.

Within weeks, Paulina began to notice subtle changes in her health. Her energy levels increased and she experienced less joint pain and inflammation.

She also noticed an improvement in my digestion and general health. Encouraged by these positive changes, she devoted herself more to her primitive lifestyle.

As time passed, the progress Paulina made became more and more noticeable.

Her symptoms continued to ease, and her autoimmune disease appeared to be in remission. It doesn't count anymore.

A raw lifestyle involves consuming foods that are uncooked, unprocessed, and in their natural state.

This type of diet is gaining popularity due to its many health benefits, including weight loss, improved digestion, increased energy levels, and reduced risk of chronic disease.

If you're interested in adopting a raw food lifestyle, Here are some tips to get you started:

1. Slow start

Switching to a raw diet can be challenging, especially if you're used to eating cooked and processed foods.

To make the transition easier, start by including more raw fruits and vegetables in your diet. You can also try substituting a cooked meal for a raw meal each day and gradually increasing the number of raw meals over time.

2. Experiment with different recipes
A raw food diet shouldn't be boring or bland. There are many fresh and nutritious recipes available online and in cookbooks. Experiment with different recipes to find the one you like best and that suits your preferences.

3. Focus on nutritious foods
Raw diets may lack some nutrients, such as protein, calcium and vitamin B12.
To make sure you get all the nutrients your body needs, focus on eating nutrient-dense foods like green leafy vegetables, nuts, seeds, and legumes.

4. Invest in quality cookware
Preparing raw meals requires special kitchen tools, such as a high-speed blender, food processor, and dehydrator. Investing in quality cookware can make preparing raw meals easier and more enjoyable.

5. Listen to your body
Like any diet, it's important to listen to your body and make any necessary adjustments. If you feel unwell or experience any negative side effects from a raw diet, consider seeing a healthcare practitioner or registered dietitian.

Adopting a raw food lifestyle can be a great way to improve your health and well-being.

6. Plan your meals

Planning your meals ahead of time can help you stick to a raw food diet and make sure you get all the nutrients you need. Make your shopping list and stock up on fresh fruits, vegetables, nuts and seeds. You can also prepare meals in advance and store them in the refrigerator or freezer for convenience.

7. Stay hydrated

Raw fruits and vegetables have a high water content, which may help you stay hydrated.
However, it is still important to drink plenty of water throughout the day to aid digestion, detoxification, and overall health.

8. Join the community

Joining the raw food community can provide support, motivation, and inspiration as you transition to a raw food lifestyle. Find local meetups, online forums, or social media groups to connect with like-minded people and share tips and recipes.

9. Practice mindful eating

Eating raw food isn't just about what you eat, it's about how you eat it. Practice mindful eating by eating slowly, savoring every bite, and paying attention to your body's hunger and satiety signals. This can help you enjoy your meal more and avoid overeating.

10. Be flexible

A raw food lifestyle isn't necessarily all or nothing. You can be flexible and incorporate cooked foods or animal products into your diet if it's best for your body and lifestyle. The most important thing is to listen to your body and make choices that support your health and well-being.

By starting slowly, experimenting with different recipes, focusing on nutrient-dense foods, investing in high-quality cooking tools, and listening to your body, you can successfully switch to a raw food diet and reap the many benefits from it.

# CHAPTER ONE

# THE POWER OF RAW

In recent years, there has been a growing interest in a raw food diet as a way to improve health and well-being.
Raw eaters believe that eating uncooked, unprocessed foods can provide the body with essential nutrients and enzymes that are lost when food is cooked.

The Power of the Raw Diet: How a Raw Diet Can Transform Your Health explores the benefits of a raw diet and how it can positively affect your physical and mental health. From losing weight to improving digestion, this book delves into the science behind a raw food diet and offers practical tips for incorporating raw foods into your daily routine. Whether you are a seasoned raw foodist or just starting out, this book is an invaluable resource for anyone looking to improve their health and vitality through natural, unrefined foods.
Raw foods have become increasingly popular in recent years, and for good reason.The power of fresh foods is undeniable as they provide numerous benefits for our health and well-being. From improving digestion to boosting energy levels, a raw food diet can change the way we feel and live.

One of the most important benefits of a raw food diet is improved digestion. Raw foods are rich in enzymes that aid in digestion, allowing our bodies to break down and absorb nutrients more easily.

This can help reduce bloating, prevent constipation, and improve overall bowel health. In addition to improving digestion, a raw food diet can also boost energy levels. Raw foods are rich in nutrients and provide the body with the energy it needs to function optimally. This can help reduce fatigue and improve overall productivity throughout the day.

Another benefit of a raw food diet is weight loss. Raw foods are naturally low in calories and high in fiber, making them a great choice for those looking to lose some extra pounds.

Unlike other diets that leave you hungry and deprived, a raw food diet can help you achieve your weight loss goals without sacrificing appetite or satisfaction. Raw foods are also known for their anti-inflammatory properties, which can help reduce inflammation in the body.

Chronic inflammation is linked to many health problems, including heart disease, cancer, and autoimmune diseases.

By incorporating more raw foods into your diet, you can reduce your risk of developing these diseases and improve your overall health.

Additionally, a raw food diet can improve skin health. Raw foods are rich in vitamins, minerals, and antioxidants that can help reduce acne, wrinkles, and other skin problems. Eating a diet rich in raw foods can help your skin look radiant and healthy.

Raw diets have also been linked to a lower risk of chronic diseases such as heart disease, diabetes and cancer.

By eating a diet rich in nutrients, you can strengthen your immune system and reduce your risk of disease. Raw foods are full of vitamins and minerals that can boost immune function.

By eating fresh foods, you can strengthen your immune system and reduce your risk of disease. Finally, raw diets have been linked to increased longevity.

By improving health and well-being through fresh foods, we can live longer, healthier lives,the power of fresh food is undeniable. A raw food diet can improve digestion, increase energy levels, aid in weight loss, reduce inflammation, improve skin health, reduce the risk of chronic disease, boost immune function, improve sleep quality and potentially increase life expectancy.

By adding more raw foods to our diet, we can improve our health and well-being.

How A Raw Food Diet Can Transform Your Health:
Raw food diet refers to the potential health benefits that can be achieved with a raw food diet. This type of diet involves consuming raw, whole, plant-based foods that are rich in nutrients and enzymes.

By eating in this way, individuals can benefit from better digestion, increase energy levels, lose weight, and reduce their risk of chronic disease.

Raw's strength lies in the transformative effect this type of diet can have on an individual's health and well-being.

1.Improves Digestion:
Fresh foods are rich in enzymes that aid digestion.Eating raw foods can improve digestion, reduce bloating, and prevent constipation.

2.Increased energy:
Raw foods are rich in nutrients and provide the body with the energy it needs to function optimally.By eating fresh foods, you can increase your energy levels and reduce fatigue.

3.Weight loss:
Fresh foods are low in calories and high in fiber, which may help you lose weight naturally.A raw food diet can help you achieve your weight loss goals without feeling deprived or hungry.

4.Reduce inflammation:
Many raw foods have anti-inflammatory properties, which can help reduce inflammation in the body. Chronic inflammation is linked to many health problems, including heart disease, cancer, and autoimmune diseases.

5.Improves skin health:
Raw foods are rich in vitamins, minerals, and antioxidants that can improve skin health.Eating

raw foods can help reduce acne, wrinkles, and other skin problems.

6. Reduce the risk of chronic diseases:
Raw diets are rich in nutrients that can help prevent chronic diseases such as heart disease, diabetes and cancer.
By eating raw foods, you can reduce your risk of developing these diseases.

7.Better mental health:
Fresh foods are rich in nutrients that promote brain health.Eating raw foods can help improve cognitive function, reduce stress, and improve overall mental health.

8.Improved immune function:
Raw foods are rich in vitamins and minerals that can boost immune function.By eating fresh foods, you can strengthen your immune system and reduce your risk of disease.

9.Sleep better:
Raw foods are rich in magnesium and other nutrients that can improve sleep quality.By eating fresh foods, you will be able to sleep better and wake up feeling refreshed.

10.Increased Longevity:
Raw food diets have been linked to increased longevity.By eating fresh foods, you can improve

your health and potentially live a longer, healthier life.
Kissing a rough lifestyle can achieve many advantages of your health and happiness.

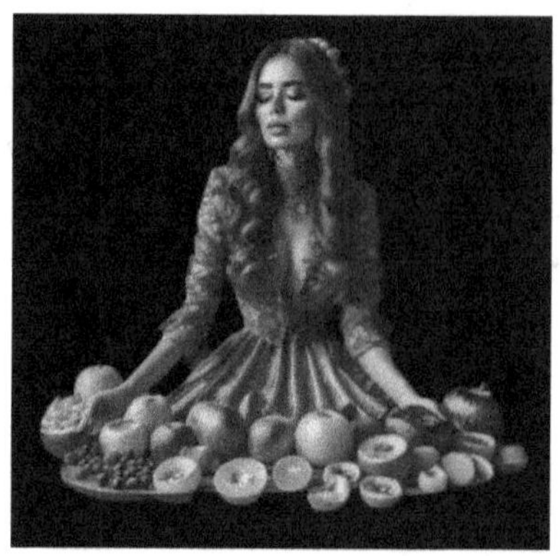

# THE BENEFITS OF EMBRACING A RAW FOOD LIFESTYLE

1. Increased energy levels
2. Improve digestion
3. Weight loss
4. Cleaner skin
5. Reduce inflammation
6. sleep better
7. Reducing the risk of chronic diseases
8. Improve mental clarity
9. Stronger immune system
10. improves mood
11. Better absorption of nutrients
12. Reducing the risk of cancer
13. Improves heart health
14. Reduction of Blood pressure
15. Reduce the risk of diabetes
16. Better gut health
17. Improve athletic performance
18. Boost hydration

19.Reduce the risk of stroke
20.Oral health improvement
21.Better Vision
22.Reducing the risk of osteoporosis
23.Increased lifespan
24.Reducing the risk of Alzheimer's disease
25.Lower cholesterol levels
26.Reducing the risk of kidney stones
27.Improves joint health
28.Reducing the risk of gallstones
29.Improve liver function
30.Reducing the risk of developing asthma
31.Enhance fertility
32.Reducing the risk of developing arthritis
33.Better menstrual hygiene
34.Reducing the risk of depression and anxiety
35.Improve respiratory health
36.Reduce the risk of allergic reactions
37.Improves hair and nail health
38.Reduces the risk of constipation and bloating
39.Promotes vitality and general health
40.Improve environmental sustainability by reducing carbon emissions and waste generation.

# RAW LIVING

## improved Health And Disease Prevention

Living the raw life, also known as the raw lifestyle, has gained popularity due to its many benefits for overall health and disease prevention. Here are some key benefits:

1. Boost your nutrient supply:
Raw foods, such as fruits, vegetables, nuts, and seeds, are full of essential vitamins, minerals, and enzymes.
By consuming these foods in their natural state, you will maximize nutrient absorption and provide your body with the essentials it needs for optimal health.

2. Improve digestion:
Raw foods are high in fiber, which aids digestion and helps maintain a healthy digestive system.
The enzymes in raw foods also promote healthy digestion, which reduces stress on the digestive system.

3. Advanced Energy Levels:
Raw foods contain natural, easily digestible sugars for a rapid and sustained release of energy.

By avoiding processed and refined foods, which can lead to an energy drain, you can benefit from improved energy levels throughout the day.

4. Weight control:
A raw food lifestyle often leads to weight loss or maintenance due to the higher fiber content and lower calorie density of raw foods.
Raw fruits and vegetables are often low in calories, making it possible to reach a healthy weight without feeling deprived.

5. Disease prevention:
Raw foods are rich in antioxidants, which help neutralize free radicals and reduce the risk of chronic diseases, including heart disease, cancer and diabetes.
In addition, the abundance of vitamins and minerals found in raw foods supports a strong immune system, making you more resistant to disease.

6. Improves skin health:
The high water content and essential nutrients in raw foods contribute to healthier, more radiant skin.
Eating raw foods has the potential to reduce common skin problems, such as acne, eczema, and dry skin.

7. Mental clarity and emotional well-being:
A raw food lifestyle often improves mental clarity and focus. Nutrient-dense foods can support brain function and provide nutrients needed for optimal

cognitive health. In addition, some people report feeling more emotionally balanced and happy.

It's important to note that while a raw food lifestyle offers many benefits, it may not be right for everyone.

You should consult with a healthcare professional or dietitian before making any significant dietary changes to ensure they meet your specific health needs and goals.

# CHAPTER TWO

## PRACTICAL TIPS FOR TRANSITIONING TO A RAW FOOD

Switching to a raw food diet can be a rewarding and health-promoting adventure.
Here are some practical tips to ease the transition:

Make a gradual change:
start with more raw fruits and vegetables in your meals, and gradually reduce cooked foods. This allows thebody to adjust to the change.

Variety is key:
Explore the wide range of raw foods available to ensure you're getting the right amount of nutrition. Include fruits, vegetables, nuts, seeds, and sprouts in your diet.

Prepare food the right way:
Invest in a good blender, juicer, and food processor to prepare delicious raw meals.
Experiment with recipes and explore different textures and flavors.

Hydrate:

Drink plenty of water and include nutritious fruits and vegetables such as cucumber and watermelon in your meals.

Research and Education:
Learn about proper nutrient formulations, seed soaking, and seed and germination techniques to improve nutrient absorption.

Eat carefully:
Chew your food well, savoring every bite. This aids digestion and allows your body to absorb the maximum amount of nutrients.

Watch your food intake:
Make sure you're getting enough protein, vitamins and minerals by consulting a dietitian or nutritionist familiar with raw food diets.

Listen to your body:
Pay attention to any changes or reactions your body feels during the transition period. Adjust your diet accordingly and seek professional advice if necessary.

Meal planning:
Plan your meals in advance to avoid last-minute temptations or reliance on cooked foods.

Enjoy the process:
Enjoy the new taste and texture of fresh food. Experiment with new recipes, join the fresh food

community, and celebrate the benefits of a healthier lifestyle.

1.Here are 30 meal planning tips:
Start by setting specific goals for your meal planning, such as eating healthy or saving money.

2.Take inventory of your pantry, refrigerator, and freezer before you plan your meals so you can use ingredients you already have on hand.

3. Plan your meals based on seasonal produce for the best taste and affordability.

4. Consider batch cooking and meal prepping to save time during the week.

5. Include a variety of food groups in your meal plan to ensure a balanced diet.

6. Experiment with new recipes and flavors to make your meals interesting.

7. Schedule weekly meals to stay organized and avoid making decisions at the last minute.

8. Plan leftovers and incorporate them into later meals to reduce waste.

9. Consider the special dietary needs or preferences of family members.

10. Pay attention to portion sizes to avoid overeating and reduce food waste.

11. Include easy meals on busy days or when you don't have much time.

12. Buy fresh and healthy fruits vegetables.

13. Make a shopping list based on your meal plan to avoid unnecessary shopping.

14. Consider using an online grocery delivery service for convenience.

15. Buy in bulk for essential components to save money in the long run.

16. Use the freezer to store pre-portioned meals or ingredients.

17. Plan meals that can be made into many different dishes to add variety.

18. Take advantage of offers and discounts when planning meals to save money.

19. Don't be afraid to simplify your meals with simple ingredients and simple recipes.

20. Cook larger portions and freeze leftovers for later use.

21. Get creative with meal planning for themed nights like Taco Tuesday or Meatless Monday.

22. Involve your family in the meal planning process to suit everyone's preferences.

23. Try planning meals using common ingredients to reduce waste and save money.

24. Use a slow cooker or pressure cooker to prepare meals quickly and easily.

25. Incorporate different cooking methods like grilling and frying to add variety to your meals.
26. Consider incorporating plant-based meals to reduce environmental impact.

27. Always stock essential ingredients such as spices, oils, and grains in the pantry.

28. Meal planning is flexible and can be adjusted based on schedule changes or unexpected events.

29. Take advantage of technology, like a meal planning app or recipe site, for inspiration and organization.

30. Allow yourself to be flexible and adaptable.

# Grocery Shopping And Food Preparation Technique

Expert advice on grocery shopping and food preparation techniques for living a raw food lifestyle

Adopting a raw food lifestyle can offer many health benefits, including increased energy levels, improved digestion, and improved nutrient intake.
However, successfully adopting and maintaining this lifestyle requires careful consideration of food preparation and procurement techniques.
In this book, we'll give you expert advice on how to make informed choices when shopping and effective food preparation techniques for raw food lovers.

I. Shop for Fresh Food And Plan Ahead:
Plan weekly meals and make detailed shopping lists. This will help you stay organized and avoid unnecessary purchases.

2.Choose fresh and organic:
Choose organic, locally sourced fruits, vegetables, and herbs whenever possible. They are free from harmful pesticides and retain maximum nutritional content.

3.Diversity issues:

Include a variety of products in your shopping cart to ensure a variety of nutrients. Experiment with different fruits and vegetables to make your meals enjoyable and balanced.

4.Maturity test:
When buying fruit, choose ripe not unripe fruit. This will ensure the optimal flavor and texture for your raw dish.

5.Stock up on the essentials:
Always stock your pantry with fresh foods like nuts, seeds, dried fruits, and superfoods like spirulina and chia seeds. These items can be used to prepare nutritious and delicious recipes.

6.Read the label:
Pay attention to labels, even for fresh food products.
Avoid ingredients such as added sugars, preservatives, and artificial additives.

# CHAPTER THREE

## Raw Food Processing Techniques

1.Wash well:
Clean all fruits and vegetables with water to remove surface dirt, bacteria or chemicals.
Use a vegetable brush if necessary, and consider using a food-grade cleaner as an extra precaution.

2. Investing in Quality Equipment:
Stock your kitchen with essentials like a high-speed blender, food processor, dehydrator, and spiralizer. These tools will make it easy to create a variety of raw recipes.

3. Soaking and germination:
Soak nuts, seeds, and beans overnight to improve digestion and activate their full nutritional potential. Germination can increase the bioavailability of nutrients.

4. Nutritional Composition:
Discover the principles of proper nutritional combinations to aid digestion.
Avoid combining starchy foods with protein and focus on pairing fruits with green leafy vegetables or non-starchy vegetables.

Green Smoothie Bowl:
Combine spinach, banana, almond milk, and a scoop of protein powder. Garnish with fresh berries, chia seeds, and sliced almonds.
Chia seed pudding:
Mix chia seeds with almond milk, vanilla extract, and a sweetener of your choice.
Leave it overnight and enjoy the fruit.

Raw vegan pancakes:
Combine ground flaxseed, mashed banana, and almond meal. Bake in a dehydrator or oven over low heat until set.

Raw Energy Bar:
Mix dates, nuts, and your favorite dried fruits. Press the mold and let it cool until it hardens. Cut it into bars and enjoy it on the go.

Avocado Toast:
Spread mashed avocado on raw bread or lettuce wraps. Garnish with tomato slices, sprouts and a pinch of sea salt.

Lunch Recipe:
Raw Pumpkin Noodles with Pesto Use a spiralizer to make zucchini noodles.
Mix it with a homemade pesto made with basil, pine nuts, garlic, and olive oil.

Raw Veggie Pack:

Wrap your favorite veggies like bell peppers, cucumbers, carrots, and avocados in large lettuce leaves. Drizzle with fragrant tahini vinegar.

Raw Nori Roll:
Fill nori sheets with chopped greens, avocado, and sprouts. Roll it tightly and cut it into small pieces. Served with tamari or coconut aminos.

Raw taco salad:
Layer of chopped lettuce, diced tomato, bell pepper, and avocado. Top with homemade cashew sour cream and sprinkle with crushed raw tortilla chips.

Raw gazpacho:
Mix ripe tomatoes, cucumbers, peppers, garlic and onions.
Add some olive oil and lemon juice. Serve cold and garnish with fresh herbs.

Dinner Recipe:
Raw Zucchini Pasta with Marinara Sauce:
Combine zucchini with pasta and toss with raw tomato marinara sauce made from mixed tomatoes, sun-dried tomatoes, herbs, and spices.

Raw Cauliflower Fried Rice:
Blend cauliflower flakes in a food processor until they resemble rice. Stir them in with chopped vegetables, tamarind, and sesame oil for a delicious and satisfying meal.

# 11 Quick And Easy Breakfast Ideas From Fresh Foods

Healthy and easy options to make the most important meals of the day extra tasty.

Breakfast should be the most important and complete meal of the day. However, with late nights and busy work schedules, you may not have enough rest, time, or energy to get ready in time. However, instead of completely ignoring it, you should at least try to make yourself a delicious breakfast! Breakfast should be eaten within two hours of waking up, which is enough to eat a bowl of fresh fruit or enjoy a fresh green juice! Not only is it quick and easy to make, but it's also very healthy! Read on to learn more about these healthy and comforting breakfast ideas that will keep you energized all day long!

## 1. Marinated Skewers:

It's a great way to start the day. The marinated skewers are lively and flavorful, which makes them perfect for any type of breakfast.

It is very easy to make, all you need are skewers and pieces of fresh organic fruit like bananas, strawberries, pineapple, apples, grapes, kiwi or any other fruit you like.

To prepare the marinade, mix the grated ginger and lemon juice, then add the maple syrup. Toss and toss with fruit skewers in the evening for a delicious breakfast.

Leaving it in the fridge overnight helps the fruit absorb the rich flavor of the marinade.

You can also make a simpler version of this recipe by chopping three to five seasonal fruits and placing them in a bowl with a little salt and lemon juice.

2. Banana Seed Bread:

To make Banana Walnut Bread, you will need 1 cup of walnuts,

3 chopped bananas,

and 1 teaspoon of vanilla extract.

Put everything in a food processor and take it out when it becomes a paste-like consistency.

Put the mixture in a bowl and add some raisins to it. Once you're done, line up small, one-inch-thick slices of bread with the dough and leave them in the dehydrator overnight.

The classic banana bread recipe is quite different from this little wonder. In addition to the healthy aspect, it also gives a feeling of satiety and energy. It's a great way to recharge in the morning and can also be used on the go.

3. Raw Oats Muesli:

Oatmeal fights cholesterol and strengthens immunity. So you'll want to eat a healthy serving of raw oatmeal muesli in the morning. Prepare the sprouted oats and put ½ cup in a bowl, followed by the milk (or nut milk made from nuts like almonds), cinnamon, diced fruit, and chopped nuts.

Add some chia seeds, maple syrup, or raw honey for more sweetness. Mix it all together and enjoy a delicious breakfast.

You can also add honey, agave syrup, stevia, brown sugar, or molasses for more sweetness.


4. Banana and Chocolate Smoothie:

Here's another quick fix that's sure to be healthy and filling, but tastes like candy!

Chop up 3 bananas and put them in a blender along with a few tablespoons of cocoa powder and a cup of nut milk.

Mix until creamy and smooth. To cool it down, you can add ice or place it in the fridge until ready to make a powerful shake.

Vegetarians can choose dairy-free milk, such as almond or nut milk, while vegans can have it with any milk.


5. Raw egg protein shake:

Raw eggs can give you salmonella, but this won't happen if you choose healthy alternatives.

Mix together 1/3 cup yogurt, 1/4 cup fresh fruit, and one egg (pasteurized eggs will kill any bacteria in them and are safer to use).

Blend for 15-20 seconds to obtain a smooth mixture.

Drink it right away, if it's not finished, store it in the refrigerator.

Leaving it will ruin it.

Eggs have many benefits because they are rich in vitamin B12, which is essential for the breakdown of carbohydrates and proteins.
Other vitamins and minerals in eggs help repair and protect body cells, and distribute good amounts of calcium to maintain strong teeth and bones.

6. Breakfast Bites
The estimated time to complete this process is less than 5 minutes! Simply cut a banana, cover it with butter (i.e. nut butter), sprinkle it with chopped walnuts and finally add the raisins.
You don't even need a bowl because you can eat them while they're being prepared.

7. Pancakes:
No-bake pancakes are a dream come true. You can enjoy the rich taste without feeling guilty as it lacks sugar and processed fats.
Cut banana slices thin and mix them with some raisins, dates and a pinch of cinnamon.
Spread the mixture over the banana slices. You can then dry them out or eat them with lots of cinnamon and a little frosting.

8.Fruit tacos:
You can use taco shells for this or make your own using romaine lettuce leaves. For garnish, cut up fruits like strawberries, bananas, and pineapples.
To prepare the glaze, you can use dark chocolate, pineapple pieces, and dried figs.

9.Banana cake:
Make a batch of delicious banana bread that you can eat every morning.
It's very simple and, again, no cooking required. Combine banana slices,
1 cup rolled oats, maple syrup, and raw nut butter in a bowl.
We form the mixture and decorate it like a biscuit with seeds and raisins.
Dry it until you are satisfied with the texture and save it as a breakfast cracker.

10. Breakfast Pudding:
This pudding is all fruit and once you eat it, you'll never use store-bought stuff again. In a food processor, chop 3 dried mangoes, then add ½ cup of fresh or frozen mangoes, 2 banana slices, and 3 dates.
Mix until thick and smooth.
Finally, put fresh fruits and grated coconut in a bowl for a delicious breakfast.

11. Open avocado sandwich
You can make avocado and tofu toast.
Take whole wheat bread and put slices of butter on top of it.
You can also add tofu pieces to it. Finally, drizzle with coconut oil mixed with your favorite spices like thyme and enjoy a healthy breakfast.

A healthy and hearty breakfast sets the tone for the day. But finding easy breakfast recipes while keeping up with your busy schedule can be a stressful task.

We've rounded up some fresh, easy, and healthy breakfast ideas to start your day.

Breakfast provides the body with energy and essential nutrients after a long sleep. Eating raw vegetables and superfoods can help maintain the nutritional value of your diet, help you lose weight, improve digestion, and give your skin a brighter complexion.

Eating fresh, unprocessed, natural, and nutrient-dense breakfast recipes can be a delicious and easy way to stay energized throughout the day. Spiced skewers, banana seed bread, raw oatmeal muesli, chocolate banana smoothie, raw egg protein shake, and breakfast snacks are some of the fresh breakfasts to try. You can also add some other options to the breakfast menu, such as tempeh, sprouts, and herbal teas. Start incorporating it into your diet today.

## Frequently Asked Questions

Can vegans eat grains?
While most cereals are made with animal ingredients, there are plant-based cereals you can try. Try to eat whole grains that are gluten-free, as

they are rich in nutrients and easy to digest. Pseudo-grains like quinoa, buckwheat, and others.

How fast can you lose weight on a raw food diet?
This can vary from person to person and depends on many factors. Consult your doctor for more information about the raw food diet.

Can I have a great breakfast every day?
Yes, you can have fresh food for breakfast every day. Remember to include a variety of fruits, vegetables, protein and healthy fats in your meals.

Are there any restrictions or foods to avoid after eating a hearty breakfast?
When eating raw foods for breakfast, it is important to avoid processed and cooked foods such as breads, cereals, cooked meats, and eggs.

Can I prepare a raw breakfast in advance?
Yes, you can make oatmeal or chia seed pudding the day before and save it for the next day.
You can also make a variety of fruit salads and vegetable juices and store them in an airtight container in the freezer.

Can I eat a hearty breakfast if I have dietary restrictions or allergies?
Yes, you can still eat a raw breakfast if you have any dietary restrictions or allergies, but be careful about the ingredients you use.

If you have a gluten intolerance, choose a gluten-free grain such as quinoa or buckwheat. People with nut allergies can choose pumpkin and sunflower seeds as good sources of protein and healthy fats.

Can I eat raw food for breakfast while traveling or eating out?
Yes, you can follow a fresh diet for breakfast, even when you are traveling or dining out. Some restaurants and cafes may offer fresh food options, but be sure to research and plan ahead.

## Key points to remember

A fruit breakfast can be a quick and nutritious option for a busy morning meal.
Raw diets have been linked to weight loss and improved health.
Shakes and desserts are energizing recipes to keep you energized all day long.
Raw foods like fruit tacos and muesli can prevent bloating and an upset stomach while providing guilt-free calories.
Start your day with a fresh vegan breakfast to fuel your body.

# Transitioning to a Raw Food Lifestyle: A Step-by-Step Guide

1. Start by including more raw fruits and vegetables in your diet.
2. Gradually reduce the amount of processed and prepared foods.
3. Experiment with different raw recipes and find the ones you like best.
4. Invest in a good blender or food processor to prepare smoothies, dips, and sauces.
5. Include a variety of raw nuts, seeds, and sprouts in your meals.
6. Focus on eating a variety of colors and textures to make sure you get all the nutrients you need.
7. Consider joining a fresh food community or finding a support group to stay motivated and inspired.
8. Listen to your body and adjust your diet if necessary to make sure you feel better.
9. Learn how to properly combine foods to improve digestion and absorption of nutrients.
10. Include fermented foods like sauerkraut and kimchi for probiotics and gut health benefits.
11. Experiment with dried fruits and vegetables for a crunchy snack option.
12. Consider incorporating superfoods like spirulina, chia seeds, and maca powder into your diet for additional nutrients.
13. Make sure you're getting enough healthy fats from sources like avocados, nuts, and seeds.

14. Don't be hard on yourself if you make mistakes and eat cooked or processed foods from time to time.
Remember, the goal is progress, not perfection.
15. Consult a healthcare practitioner or dietitian before making any major dietary changes.

**BREAKFAST**

**Recipe Day 1:**
**Chia Pudding**

Chia pudding is a great source of healthy fats, fiber, and protein to start your day. You can also experiment with adding different flavors and toppings to change things up.
- Chia Pudding (chia seeds, almond milk, vanilla extract, maple syrup) topped with sliced banana and chopped walnuts.

Method Of Preparation
_In a bowl, mix together chia seeds, almond milk, vanilla extract, and maple syrup.
_Let it sit in the fridge overnight or for at least 4 hours until it thickens.
_Top with sliced banana and chopped walnuts before serving.

**Estimated Meal Time And Serve Time**

Prep Time   5_10 Minutes
Serve Time  Immediate or Serve Cold the next day.


## Nutritional Facts (approx)

Calories  138
Protein  4g
Carbohydrates  15g
Fiber  10g
Fat 8g
Sugar  5g

Note: Nutritional Values may vary depending on the specific ingredients used in the recipe.


## Health Benefits


Chia pudding is healthy breakfast options that offer many health benefits. Here are some of the main benefits of each:

Chia pudding:
1.Rich in fiber:
Chia seeds are a rich source of fiber, which can help support digestion and help you feel full.
2.Rich in Omega-3 Fatty Acids:

Chia seeds are one of the best sources of plant-based omega-3 fatty acids, which have been linked to improved heart health and brain function.
3.Low Sugar:
Chia pudding is naturally low in sugar, making it a good choice for those looking to reduce their sugar intake.
4.Gluten Free:
Chia seeds are naturally gluten free, making them a great choice for those with celiac disease or a gluten intolerance.

## Recipe Day 2:
## Overnight Oats

- Overnight Oats (rolled oats, almond milk, chia seeds, cinnamon, maple syrup) topped with sliced strawberries and almond butter.

Method Of Preparation
_In a jar, mix together rolled oats, almond milk, chia seeds, cinnamon, and maple syrup.
_Let it sit in the fridge overnight.
_Top with sliced strawberries and a dollop of almond butter before serving.

### Estimated Meal Time And Serve Time

Prep Time  5_10 Minutes
Serve Time  Immediate or Serve cold the next day

**Nutritional Facts (approx)**
Calories 300
Protein  11g
Carbohydrates  45g
Fiber  7g
Fat 8g
Sugar 18g

## Health Benefits

Overnight oatmeal:
1.High in fiber:
Overnight oats are also high in fiber, which aids digestion and helps you feel full.
2. Lowers cholesterol:
Oats contain a type of soluble fiber called beta-glucan, which helps lower cholesterol levels.
3. Rich in Antioxidants:
Oats are a good source of antioxidants, which can help protect against oxidative stress and inflammation in the body.
 EASY TO MAKE:
Overnight oats are a convenient breakfast option that can be made the night before, making them a great option for busy mornings.


**Recipe Day 3**
**Acai Bowl**

- Acai Bowl (frozen acai puree, mixed berries, banana, almond milk) topped with granola and coconut flakes.

Method Of Preparation
_In a blender, blend together frozen acai puree, mixed berries, banana, and almond milk until smooth.
_Pour into a bowl and top with granola and coconut flakes before serving.

### Estimated Meal Time And Serve Time

Prep Time   5_10Minutes
Serve Time   10_15 Minutes

### Nutritional Facts (approx)

Calories  250_400
Protein  3_8 grams
Carbohydrates 30_50 grams
Fiber  5_10 grams
Fat  10_20 grams
Sugar 15_30 grams

### Health Benefits

1.Acai berries are rich in antioxidants, which can help protect the body from free radical damage.

2.They are also a good source of fiber, healthy fats, and vitamins and minerals such as vitamin C, vitamin A, and calcium.

3.Chia seeds are also high in fiber and healthy fats, as well as protein, calcium and magnesium.

4.They are also a good source of antioxidants and can help support healthy digestion.

5. Acai bowls can be nutritious additions to a balanced diet.

**Recipe Day 4**
**Vegan Chia Pudding**

Ingredients
- 1/2 cup chia seeds
2 cups almond milk (or any plant-based milk of your choice)
1-2 tablespoons of maple syrup (optional)
_1 teaspoon of vanilla extract
Fresh fruits and nuts for garnish

Method Of Preparation
1. In a bowl, mix the chia seeds, almond milk, maple syrup (if using), and vanilla extract.
2. Stir well and leave for at least 30 minutes or overnight in the fridge until the mixture thickens and resembles pudding.
3. Garnish with fresh fruits and nuts to your liking and enjoy!

**Estimated Meal Time And Serve Time**

Prep Time  5_10 Minutes
Serve Time  10_15 Minutes

## Nutrition Facts (approx)

Calories  150_200
Protein  4_6 grams
Carbohydrates  20_25 grams
Fiber  10_12 grams
Fat  7_10 grams
Sugar  0_5 grams

## Health Benefits

Vegan chia pudding
which can help protect the body from free radical damage. They are also a good source of fiber, healthy fats, and vitamins and minerals such as vitamin C, vitamin A, and calcium.
Chia seeds are also high in fiber and healthy fats, as well as protein, calcium and magnesium. They are also a good source of antioxidants and can help support healthy digestion.

## Recipe Day 5
## Raw Food Breakfast Bowl

A raw breakfast can be both nutritious and delicious. Here is a simple, easy and nutritious breakfast recipe:

Ingredients
- 1 banana
- A cup of mixed berries (strawberry, blueberry, raspberry)
- 1/4 cup of raw almonds
- 1 teaspoon of chia seeds
- 1 teaspoon of raw honey
- 1/2 cup coconut water
- 1/2 teaspoon cinnamon

Methods Of Preparation
1.Start by soaking raw almonds overnight in water. This will help soften it and make it easier to digest.
2. In the morning, take out the almonds and wash them.
3. Place the almonds, bananas, mixed berries, chia seeds, raw honey, and cinnamon in a blender.
4. Pour in the coconut water and mix until smooth.
5. Pour the mixture into a bowl and serve immediately. This ready-to-eat breakfast is full of nutrients. Bananas and mixed berries are a good source of vitamins and antioxidants.
Raw almonds are a great source of healthy fats and protein, while chia seeds are a good source of fiber. Pure honey adds sweetness without the need for refined sugar, and cinnamon provides a delicious flavor while helping to regulate blood sugar levels.
Coconut water provides hydration and electrolytes. This breakfast is not only healthy, but also delicious and satisfying.

## Estimated Meal Time And Serve Time

Prep Time 10_15 Minutes
Serve Time  Immediate


## Nutritional Facts (approx)

However, here are some approximate nutritional values for common ingredients that can be used in raw breakfast bowls:

Raw oats (half cup):
150 calories, 5g protein, 27g carbs, 4g fiber, 3g fat, 1g sugar.
Chia seeds (1 tablespoon):
60 calories, 2g protein, 5g carbs, 5g fiber, 4g fat, 0g sugar.
Flaxseeds (1 tablespoon):
37 calories, 1g protein, 2g carbs, 2g fiber, 3g fat, 0g sugar.
Almond milk (1 cup):
60-80 calories, 1-2g protein, 1-8g carbs, 0-1g fiber, 2-7g fat, 0-7g sugar
Fresh fruit (1 cup):
varies by fruit, but generally ranges from 50 to 150 calories, with varying amounts of protein, carbohydrates, fiber, and sugar.


## Health Benefits

This breakfast smoothie bowl contains many health benefits, including:

1. Rich in nutrients:
The juice bowl is made of fresh fruits, vegetables, and nuts, all of which are rich in essential nutrients such as vitamins, minerals, and antioxidants.

2. Boosts Energy:
The combination of fruits and nuts in this smoothie bowl provides a quick boost of energy, making it the perfect breakfast option for those who need to jump-start their day.

3. Promotes digestive health: The fiber found in fruits and vegetables helps support healthy digestion and prevent constipation.

4. Promotes Weight Loss: This smoothie bowl is low in calories and high in fiber, making it an ideal breakfast option for those looking to lose weight.

5. Boosts immunity:
Antioxidants found in fruits and vegetables help strengthen the immune system, thus protecting the body from diseases and infections.

6. Improve Skin Health:
The nutrients in this juice bowl help promote healthy skin, which reduces the appearance of wrinkles and other signs of aging.

All in all, this breakfast smoothie bowl is a delicious and nutritious way to start your day, providing you with many health benefits that will help you feel energized and healthy throughout the day.

<h1 style="text-align:center">LUNCH</h1>

Here Are 5 Raw Food Lunch Recipes That You Can Try


**Recipe Day 1**
**Vegan vegetarian food**

Ingredients
4 large green cabbage leaves
- 1 mashed avocado
- 1/2 cup chopped cucumber
- 1/2 cup chopped sweet pepper
- 1/4 cup chopped red onion
- 1/4 cup chopped fresh cilantro
Juice of 1 lemon
- Salt and pepper to taste

Method Of Preparation
Firstly, Wash and dry the cabbage, then remove the tough stems.
2. In a bowl, mix the mashed avocado, cucumber, bell pepper, red onion, cilantro, lime juice, salt, and pepper.
3. Sprinkle the mixture over the collard greens and roll it up nicely, like a burrito. Cut it in half and enjoy!

**Estimated Meal Time And Serve Time**
Prep Time  20_30 Minutes
Serve Time  immediate

**Nutritional Facts (approx)**

Calories  200
Protein  5_10 grams
Carbohydrates  20_50 grams
Fiber 5_10 grams
Fat  10_20 grams
Sugar  5_10 grams

## HEALTH BENEFITS

There are many health benefits associated with eating Vegan Vegetarian food.

1. Rich in Nutrients:

This dish is full of essential vitamins and minerals, including vitamin C, potassium, and fiber, which are important for maintaining good health.

2. Low in calories:

Vegetables, are low in calories and high in fiber, making them a great choice for weight management.

3. Rich in Antioxidants:

The vegetables sauce used in this dish contains antioxidants that help protect the body from damage caused by free radicals.

4. Good for digestion:

The fiber content in vegetables promotes healthy digestion and prevents constipation.

5. Promotes Heart Health: Vegetarian diets have been shown to reduce the risk of heart disease and stroke, and this dish is a great example of a heart-healthy meal.

Overall, eating vegan vegetarian food provides many health benefits while still being delicious and satisfying.


**Recipe Day 2**
**Vegetable Zucchini Noodles With Pesto**

Ingredients
2 medium sized butternut squash, rolled into noodles
- 1/2 cup fresh basil leaves
- 1/4 cup of pine nuts
- 1 clove of garlic
- 1/4 cup of olive oil
- Salt and pepper to taste

Method Of Preparation
1. Roll the zucchini into noodles and set aside.
2. Put the basil, pine nuts, garlic, olive oil, salt, and pepper in a food processor. pulse until smooth.
3. Mix zucchini noodles with pesto and enjoy.

**Estimated Meal Time And Serve Time**
Prep Time 1_2 Minutes
Serve Time  Immediate / keep in the fridge

**Nutritional Facts (approx)**
Calories   200_300
Protein   5_10 grams
Carbohydrates   20_30 grams
Fiber   5_10 grams

Fat 10_20 grams
Sugar 5_10 grams

## HEALTH BENEFITS

There are many health benefits associated with Vegetable Zucchini noodles with pesto
Firstly,  Rich in Nutrients:
This dish is full of essential vitamins and minerals, including vitamin C, potassium, and fiber, which are important for maintaining good health.
2.Low-calorie:
Vegetables, especially zucchini, are low in calories and high in fiber, making them a great choice for weight management.
3. Rich in Antioxidants:
The pesto sauce used in this dish contains antioxidants that help protect the body from damage caused by free radicals.
4. Good for Digestion:
The fiber content in vegetables helps promote healthy digestion and prevent constipation.
5. Promotes Heart Health: Vegetarian diets have been shown to reduce the risk of heart disease and stroke, and this dish is a great example of a heart-healthy meal.
Overall, eating vegan and vegan zucchini noodles with pesto can provide many health benefits while still being delicious and satisfying.

It should be noted that this dish is generally low in calories and high in fiber, making it a great choice for those looking to control weight or improve digestion.
Alternatively, the protein content can be increased by adding tofu, chickpeas, or other plant-based protein sources.


**Recipe Day 3**
**Vegetarian Carrot and Ginger Soup**
Ingredients
- 4 cups of chopped carrots
- 1/2 cup chopped onion
- 2 garlic cloves
- 2 tablespoons of fresh ginger, finely chopped
- 4 cups of vegetable broth
- Salt and pepper

Method Of Preparation
1. In a blender or food processor, puree the carrots, onions, garlic, ginger, and vegetable stock until smooth.
2. Season with salt and pepper to taste.
3. Chill the soup in the refrigerator for at least 30 minutes before serving.

**Estimated Meal Time And Serve Time**

Prep Time 20_30 Minutes
Serve Time   Immediate

## Nutritional Facts (approx)

Calories  200
Protein  5_10 grams
Carbohydrates  20_30 grams
Fiber   5_10 grams
Fat 10_20 grams
Sugar 5_10 grams

## Health Benefits

1. Rich in nutrients:
Carrots are an excellent source of vitamin A, while ginger is rich in antioxidants and has anti-inflammatory properties.
2. May improve digestion:
Ginger has been shown to aid digestion and reduce nausea.
3. May support the immune system: Vitamin A in carrots can help support immune function.
4. Low in calories:
This soup is generally low in calories, which makes it a great choice for those looking to control their weight.

**Recipe Day 4**
**Raw Vegan Rainbow Salad**
Ingredients

2 cups shredded romaine lettuce
- 1 cup shredded red cabbage
- 1 cup chopped cabbage
- 1/2 cup chopped carrots
- 1/2 cup chopped cucumber
- 1/2 cup chopped sweet pepper
- 1/2 cup chopped cherry tomatoes
- A quarter cup of chopped fresh parsley
Juice of 1 lemon
- Salt and pepper to taste

Method Of Preparation
Firstly,  In a large bowl, combine romaine lettuce, red cabbage, kale, carrots, cucumber, bell pepper, cherry tomatoes, and parsley.
2. Pour in the lemon juice and season with salt and pepper to taste.

## Estimated Meal Time And Serve Time

Prep Time 5_10Minutes
Serve Time  Immediate

Nutritional Facts (approx)
Calories 60
Protein  2grams
Carbohydrates  8grams
Fiber  3 grams
Fat 3grams
Sugar 4grams

## Health Benefits

1. Rich in nutrients:

This salad is made with a variety of colorful vegetables that provide a variety of vitamins and minerals.

2. Rich in fiber:

The high fiber content can help improve digestion and promote satiety.

3. May support heart health:

The vegetables in this salad are often low in fat and rich in antioxidants, which can help support heart health.

4. Low Calories:

This salad is generally low in calories, which makes it a great choice for those looking to control their weight.


**Recipe Day 5**
**Raw Vegan Cauliflower Fried Rice**

Ingredients

1 head of cauliflower, cut into pieces like rice

- 1/2 cup chopped sweet pepper

- 1/2 cup chopped onion

- 1/2 cup of chopped broccoli

- A quarter cup of tamari or soy sauce

- 2 tablespoons of sesame oil

- 2 minced garlic cloves


Method Of Preparation

1. In a large skillet, heat the sesame oil over medium-high heat.
2. Add garlic cloves and fry  for 1 minute.
3. Add the cauliflower rice, bell pepper, onion and broccoli, saute for 5-7 minutes until the vegetables are soft.
4. Add tamari or soy sauce and mix. Eat hot.

## Estimated Meal Time And Serve Time

Prep Time 15_30 Minutes
Serve Time Immediate


Nutritional Facts (approx)
Calories 100_150 calories
Protein 2_4 grams
Carbohydrates
Fiber  3_5 grams
Fat 5_8 grams
Sugar 2_4 grams


## Health Benefits

A Raw Vegetable Rainbow Salad Is A colorful and nutritious side dish that often includes a variety of vegetables, fruits, nuts, and seeds. Among the health benefits of this dish are the following:

1.Rich In Fiber:

This raw vegetable rainbow trout salad is rich in fiber, which can help support healthy digestion and prevent constipation.

2. Full Of Vitamins And Minerals:

The colorful fruits and vegetables in this dish provide a variety of vitamins and minerals, including vitamin C, vitamin A, potassium and folate.

3. Low Calorie:

Since this dish is mainly composed of fruits and vegetables that are low in calories, it can be a great option for those looking to maintain or lose weight.

4. Rich in Antioxidants:

Most of the ingredients in this dish are rich in antioxidants, which can help protect the body from free radical damage and reduce the risk of chronic diseases.

5. Control blood sugar:

The high fiber content in raw vegetable rainbow salad can also help regulate blood sugar, making it a good choice for people with diabetes or insulin resistance.

It is important to note that the actual time taken to prepare these meals can vary depending on each individual's preferences and cooking skills. In addition, some recipes may require additional ingredients or steps that may increase preparation time.

You should read the recipe carefully before you start to make sure you have all the ingredients and equipment you need, and plan to add the time accordingly.

**DINNER**
**Recipe Day 1**
**Raw Zucchini Pasta With Avocado Pesto**
Ingredients
2-3 medium zucchini
2 ripe avocados
1 cup fresh basil leaves
1/2 cup fresh spinach leaves
1/4 cup of pine nuts
2 cloves of garlic
2 tablespoons of lemon juice
2 tablespoons pure extra
olive oil
Salt and pepper to taste
Garnish options: cherry tomatoes, pepper slices, olives or sprouts.

Method Of Preparation
Use a spiral peeler or slicer to prepare zucchini noodles.
Keep them in a bowl. In a food processor, combine avocado, basil, spinach, pine nuts, garlic, lemon juice, olive oil,
salt, and pepper.
Mix until smooth and creamy.
Pour avocado pesto over zucchini noodles, tossing until evenly coated.
Leave the dish to steep for 10 to 15 minutes for the flavors to meld.

Serve the zucchini noodles with your choice of toppings, such as cherry tomatoes, pepper slices, olives, or sprouts.
Enjoy raw zucchini noodles with avocado pesto! It's a refreshing, nutrient-dense meal that's perfect for a primal lifestyle.

### Estimated Meal Time And Serve Time
Prep Time  15_30 Minutes
Serve Time  Immediate


### Nutritional Facts (approx)

Calories  250 calories per serving
Protein  5 grams
Carbohydrates  15 grams
Fiber  10 grams
Fat  20 grams
Sugar  4 grams

### Health Benefits

Raw zucchini noodles with avocado pesto offer a number of health benefits thanks to the nutritional ingredients.Here are some of the benefits:
1 Rich in nutrients:
Zucchini is rich in vitamins A, C, and K, as well as minerals like potassium and manganese. Avocados are high in healthy fats, fiber, and vitamins E, K, and C.
2 Weight control:

Raw zucchini noodles are low in calories and carbohydrates, making them suitable for those watching their weight. The high fiber content helps you feel full for longer.

3 Rich in Antioxidants:

Zucchini and avocado are excellent sources of antioxidants, which help protect the body from harmful free radicals and reduce inflammation. 4 4 Heart health:

Avocados are a good source of monounsaturated fats. , which may help improve heart health by lowering levels of bad cholesterol and reducing the risk of heart disease.

5 Digestive health:

Raw zucchini noodles are high in water and fiber, which aids digestion and supports a healthy digestive system. Avocado also contains fiber, which helps promote regular bowel movements.

6 Eye health:

Zucchini is rich in vitamin A and antioxidants like lutein and zeaxanthin, which are beneficial for eye health and may help reduce the risk of age-related macular degeneration.

8 Skin health:

The combination of zucchini and avocado provides beneficial vitamins and antioxidants that help maintain healthy skin, boost collagen production, and fight skin damage caused by free radicals.

Remember that although raw zucchini pasta with avocado pesto may have health benefits, it is important to maintain a balanced diet and take into account everyone's dietary needs and preferences.

**Recipe Day 2
Raw Vegan Sushi Rolls:**

These sushi rolls are made with nori leaves, raw vegetables like cucumber, avocado, and carrots, and a variety of vegan sauces like tahini or spicy mayonnaise. It's a delicious and hearty dinner option.

Ingredients
- 2 cups of cauliflower rice
- 4 sheets of nori seaweed
- 1 avocado, cut into slices
- 1/2 cup grated carrot
- 1/2 cup chopped cucumber
- 1/2 cup chopped sweet pepper
- 1/4 cup chopped green onions
- 1 tablespoon sesame
- Tamari or soy sauce for dipping

Method Of Preparation
1. Rinse the nori sheets and place them on a flat surface.
2. Spread a layer of cauliflower rice on each sheet, leaving about 1 inch of space on top.
3. Arrange the avocado, carrots, cucumber, pepper and green onions in a single row in the center of each sheet.
4. Sprinkle the sesame seeds over the vegetables.

5. Roll the sushi tightly, starting at the bottom and use the space at the top to tape the roll.
6. Cut the sushi rolls into small pieces and serve with tamari or soy sauce for dipping.

## Nutritional Facts (approx)

Calories: 190
Fat: 10 grams
Carbohydrates: 23 grams
Fiber: 9 grams
Protein: 8 grams

## Estimated Meal Time And Serve Time

Prep Time  30_50 grams
Serve Time   Immediate

## Health Benefits:

1. Low Calorie:
Raw vegetarian sushi rolls are low in calories, making them a great choice for those looking to maintain or lose weight.
2. Rich in fiber:
Cauliflower rice and the vegetables in this dish are high in fiber, which helps promote healthy digestion and prevent constipation.
3. Rich in vitamins and minerals:
The vegetables in this dish provide a variety of vitamins and minerals, including vitamin C, vitamin A, potassium, and folate.

4. Healthy Fats:

The avocado in this dish provides healthy fats that can help improve heart health and reduce inflammation.

5. Control blood sugar:

The high fiber content in this dish can also help regulate blood sugar, making it a good choice for people with diabetes or insulin resistance.


**Recipe Day 3**
**Raw Vegetarian Pad Thai:**

This dish can be made using raw zucchini noodles as a base and topped with a homemade raw peanut sauce made with peanut butter, lime juice, tamarind, and ginger.

Add raw vegetables like bean sprouts, carrots, and bell peppers for a complete meal.

This dish can be made using raw zucchini noodles as a base and topped with a homemade raw peanut sauce made with peanut butter, lime juice, tamarind, and ginger.

Add raw vegetables such as bean sprouts, carrots, and bell peppers to mix them well.

Ingredients
- 2 medium-sized zucchini, spiralized
- 1 large spiral carrot
- 1 chopped hot red pepper
- 1/2 cup of beans

- 1/4 cup crushed pistachio
- 1/4 cup chopped coriander
- 1 lemon cut into slices

For the sauce:
- 1/4 cup of almond butter
2 tablespoons of tamari sauce
- 2 tablespoons of apple cider vinegar
- 1 tablespoon of maple syrup
- 1 minced garlic clove
- 1 teaspoon ground ginger
- 1/4 cup of water

Method Of Preparation
1. In a small bowl, whisk all sauce ingredients until smooth.
2. In a large bowl, mix the zucchini, carrots, bell peppers, and bean sprouts.
3. Pour the sauce over the vegetables and stir to combine.
4. Divide the pad Thai into bowls and garnish with chopped peanuts, cilantro and lemon wedges.

This Raw Thai Vegan pad is a great source of fiber, vitamins and minerals. Zucchini and carrots are low in calories and rich in fiber and vitamin C.
Bell peppers are also rich in vitamin C, while bean sprouts provide vitamin K and folate.
Almond butter is a good source of healthy fats and protein, while peanuts add more protein and flavor.

**Estimated Meal Time And Serving Time:**

Prep Time 20_30 Minutes
Serve Time   Immediate


**Nutritional Facts ( approx)**

Calories 150
Protein  5 grams
Carbohydrates  15 grams
Fiber  4 grams
Fat  9 grams
Sugar  7g


## Health benefits:
This raw vegan pad thai is a great choice for those looking for a healthy and delicious meal. They are low in calories, high in fiber, and packed with vitamins and minerals.
The almond and peanut butter provide healthy fats and protein, while the vegetables add plenty of nutrients to the dish. The sauce is also made with healthy ingredients and contains no added sugar or preservatives.


**Recipe Day 4**
**Raw vegan pizza:**

Raw vegan pizza can be made using cauliflower peel or flaxseed and topped with raw tomato sauce, vegetables like mushrooms and peppers, and vegan cheeses made with nuts or seeds.

Raw vegan pizza

ingredients
1 large cauliflower (homemade or store-bought)
- 1/2 cup of ketchup
1/4 cup sliced black olives
1/4 cup sliced mushrooms
- 1/4 cup chopped hot pepper
- 1/4 cup chopped red onion
- 1/4 cup chopped fresh basil
- 1 tablespoon of nutritional yeast
- Salt and pepper to taste

Method Of Preparation
1. Preheat the oven to 375 degrees Fahrenheit.
2. Drizzle the tomato sauce over the cauliflower skins.
3. Garnish with black olives, mushrooms, peppers and red onions.
4. Sprinkle with nutritional yeast, salt, and pepper.
5. Bake for 15-20 minutes or until the crust is crispy and the topping is evenly heated through.
6.Garnish with fresh basil before serving.

**Nutritional Facts (approx)**
Calories: 180
Fat: 6 grams

Carbohydrates: 25 grams
Fiber: 10 grams
Protein: 9 grams

**Estimated Meal Time And Serve Time**
Prep Time 30 Minutes
Serve Time Immediate

## Health Benefits:

1. Low-calorie:
Raw vegan pizza is a low-calorie option that can help with weight control.
2. High in fiber:
Cauliflower peels and vegetable toppings are high in fiber, which can promote healthy digestion and prevent constipation.
3. Full of vitamins and minerals:
The vegetables in this dish provide a variety of vitamins and minerals, including vitamin C, vitamin A, potassium, and folate.
4. Suitable for Vegetarians:
This dish is completely vegetarian, so it is suitable for vegetarians.
5. Control Blood Sugar:
The high fiber content of this dish can also help regulate blood sugar, making it a good choice for people with diabetes or insulin resistance.

**Recipe Day 5**

## Raw Vegan Tacos

Ingredients
- 1 head of lettuce, separated
- 1 cup tomato paste
- 1 cup chopped hot pepper
- 1/2 cup chopped red onion
- 1/2 cup chopped coriander
- 1 avocado, cut into slices
1/2 cup raw cashews, soaked in water
- 1 teaspoon of chili powder
- 1 teaspoon of dill
- 1/2 teaspoon of chili powder
- Salt and pepper to taste

Method Of Preparation
1. Place the soaked cashews in a food processor, and blend with the chili powder, cumin, paprika, salt, and pepper until smooth.
2. Arrange the lettuce leaves on a plate and add the chopped tomatoes, peppers, red onions, cilantro and avocado slices to each leaf.
3. Sprinkle cashew crumbs over each taco and serve immediately.

### Estimated Meal Time And Serve Time

Prep Time  30_45 Minutes
Serve Time Immediate

### Nutritional Facts (approx)
Calories: 320

Fat: 23 grams
Carbohydrates: 22 grams
Fiber: 10 grams
Protein: 9 grams

### Health Benefits:

1. Rich in fiber:
The lettuce leaves in this dish are rich in fiber, which helps support healthy digestion and prevents constipation.
2. Rich in vitamins and minerals:
The vegetables in this dish provide a variety of vitamins and minerals, including vitamin C, vitamin A, potassium, and folate.
3. Healthy Fats:
The avocado and cashews in this dish provide healthy fats that can help improve heart health and reduce inflammation.
4. Rich in antioxidants:
The vegetables in this dish are rich in antioxidants, which can help protect the body from free radical damage and reduce the risk of chronic diseases.
5. Control Blood Sugar:
The high fiber content of this dish can also help regulate blood sugar, making it a good choice for people with diabetes or insulin resistance.

## SNACKS

Here are 10 delicious snacks that fit into a healthy lifestyle:

1.Fresh Fruit Salad:
Combine a variety of chopped or sliced fruits like berries, watermelon, grapes, and citrus for a refreshing and nutritious snack.

2 Raw Veggie Sticks with Dipping Sauce:
Enjoy crunchy veggies like carrots, celery, peppers, and cucumbers with a delicious dipping sauce made with avocado, tahini, or nut butter.

3 Raw Energy Bars:
Make your own raw energy bars using ingredients like dates, nuts, seeds, and dried fruits. Mix them together and shape them into bars for a quick and satisfying snack.

4 Raw nuts and seeds:
Almonds, walnuts, cashews, pumpkin seeds, and sunflower seeds are all great options for a fresh snack. It is full of healthy fats, proteins and various foodstuffs.

5 Zucchini or Cucumber rolls :
Cut zucchini or cucumber along the smooth strips and wrap them with decoration such as Houmous, Guacamole or smooth vegetables.
In cutting the size of the bite, throw it with olive oil, salt and your favorite spices, then dry until you are wavy for a nutritional snack.

6 Chia seed pudding:

Mix the chia seeds with your choice of vegetative milk and let them rest until they absorb liquid seeds and create a tissue similar to candy. Add fruits or nuts to an additional and brittle flavor.

Form the mixture into small balls and refrigerate for a delicious and invigorating snack.

7 Raw Chocolate Avocado Mousse: Mix ripe avocado, raw cacao powder, a sweetener like maple syrup or dates, and a pinch of salt for a rich, creamy chocolate spread. Remember that even though these snacks are raw, they can still be eaten in moderation as part of a balanced diet.

Have fun experimenting with different flavors and ingredients!

## HEALTH BENEFITS

1. Helps maintain energy levels throughout the day
2. Provides a quick source of nutrients and vitamins
3. Overeating during meals can be avoided
4. Helps control blood sugar
5. It helps in losing and controlling weight
6. Increase variety in your diet
7. Helps meet the recommended daily intake of fruits and vegetables
8. Offers a healthy alternative to processed snacks
9. Improves digestion and gut health
10. It can strengthen the immune system
11. Improves skin health and appearance
12. It can reduce inflammation in the body

13. It improves mental clarity and focus

14. It improves mood and general health

15. This reduces the risk of chronic diseases such as heart disease and diabetes.

16. Improves athletic performance and recovery

17. It promotes healthy aging

18. It reduces the risk of nutritional deficiencies

19. It's a fun and creative way to experiment with new recipes and flavors.

20. Help create a sustainable and environmentally friendly lifestyle by reducing waste from packaged snacks.

## SMOOTHIES

Day 1:
- Green goddess juice (spinach, turnip, banana, pineapple, almond milk)

Bliss juice (blueberries, banana, chia seeds, coconut water)
- Mango Tango juice (mango, pineapple, ginger, turmeric, coconut milk)
- Fabricated berries (berries, bananas, almond butter, almond milk)
- juice with peanut butter chocolate (cocoa powder, peanut butter, banana, today, almond milk)

Day 2:
- Banana juice strawberry (strawberry, banana, coconut water)

- tropical juice at sunrise (mango, pineapple, orange juice, coconut milk)
- Blastie Berry Blast (mixed berries, bananas, almond milk)
Coconut juice with pineapple (pineapple, coconut milk, today)
- Hardi Khokhi juice (dow, bananas, almond milk)

Day 3:
Mint option juice (cucumber, mint leaves, apples, lemon juice)
- Smoot Smoothie (carrots, ginger roots, orange juice)
Radish juice (radish, mixed berries, almond milk)
Green tea juice (green chic tea powder, banana, almond milk)
Lime to watermelon (watermelon, lemon juice, coconut water)

Day 4
Avocado juice (lawyer, mango, spinach, almond milk)
- Cherry chocolate juice (cherry, cocoa powder, almond mixlwith Orange cream (orange juice, vanilla extract, coconut milk)
- Pina Colada juice (pineapple, coconut milk, history))
- A apple cake hot (apple, cinnamon, nutmeg, almond milk)

Day 5:

- juice with peanut butter and gel (peanut butter, mixed berries, almond milk)

Green monster juice (spinach, bananas, pineapple, coconut water)

Chocolate juice (cocoa powder, banana, almond milk)

- Mango Lassi juice (mango, yogurt, cardamom, almond milk)

Lemon lemon juice (wild grapes, lemon juice, almond milk)

## HEALTH BENEFITS

1. Provides a quick and convenient source of nutrients and vitamins
2. Help control blood sugar
3. It help with weight loss and control
4. Increase variety in your diet
5. Help meet the recommended daily intake of fruits and vegetables
6. Offers a healthy alternative to processed drinks
7. Improve digestion and gut health
8. It can strengthen the immune system
9. Improve skin health and appearance
10. It reduce inflammation in the body
11. It improve mental clarity and focus
12 Improve mood and general health
13. Reduce the risk of chronic diseases such as heart disease and diabetes
14. Improve athletic performance and recovery
15. It promote healthy aging
16. It reduce the risk of nutritional deficiencies

17. It can be a fun and creative way to try new recipes and flavors
18. It can help create a sustainable, eco-friendly lifestyle by reducing waste from bottled beverages.
19. It is easily customized to suit individual dietary needs and preferences
20. It is a convenient meal replacement option for busy people
21. It is a refreshing and replenishing drink in hot weather or after a workout
22. It provide a source of healthy fats with added ingredients like butter or nut butter
23. It is a source of protein by adding ingredients such as protein powder or Greek yogurt
24. It is a source of fiber with added ingredients like chia seeds or flaxseeds
25. It is a source of antioxidants by adding ingredients such as berries or dark green leafy vegetables
26. A source of calcium through added ingredients such as almond milk or kale
27 A source of iron by adding ingredients such as spinach or pumpkin seeds
28. It Is a source of vitamin C by adding its ingredients such as citrus fruits or kiwi
29. A source of vitamin E through the addition of ingredients such as almonds or sunflower seeds
30. A source of potassium by adding ingredients such as bananas or coconut water.

# Easy To Make Dishes That Can Be Prepared With Common Ingredients

Eating healthy and delicious meals doesn't have to be complicated or expensive.

With just a few simple ingredients, you can create easy and delicious dishes that will satisfy your cravings and nourish your body.

We are going to share with you some of our favorite recipes that can be made with common ingredients that you probably already have in your pantry.

**BREAKFAST:**

Firstly. Avocado Toast:
Toast a slice of whole wheat bread and spread grated butter on top. Sprinkle salt, pepper and red pepper. Add a fried egg or a slice of tomato for more flavour.

2. Greek Yogurt Parfait:
Place Greek yogurt, fresh berries, granola, and honey in a bowl or bowl. Garnish with chopped nuts or seeds for crunch.

3. Banana Cake:
Mash a ripe banana in a bowl and mix it with 2 eggs, 1/4 cup flour and a pinch of baking powder. Cook the dough in a non-stick frying pan until

golden. Served with maple syrup and banana slices.

**LUNCH:**

1. Green Bean Salad:
Drain and rinse a can of green beans and mix with chopped cucumber, tomato, red onion, and parsley. Season with lemon juice, olive oil, salt and pepper.

2. Grilled cheese sandwich:
Butter two slices of bread and place a slice of cheese between them. Bake in the skillet until the cheese melts and the bread is crispy.

3. Quinoa bowl:
Cook quinoa according to package directions and mix with roasted vegetables (like sweet potatoes, zucchini, and bell peppers), avocado, and feta cheese. Drizzle with balsamic vinegar and olive oil .

**DINNER:**

1.Pasta in Tomato Sauce:
Cook spaghetti according to package directions and combine with canned tomato sauce, garlic, onion, and basil. Garnish with grated parmesan.

2. Grilled Salmon:
Season the salmon fillets with salt, pepper and lemon juice. Bake in the oven at 400 degrees

Fahrenheit for 15 to 20 minutes, until cooked through. Served with steamed vegetables.

3. Stir-fry:
Heat the oil in a wok or wok and sauté sliced chicken, beef, or tofu with chopped vegetables (such as broccoli, carrots, and bell peppers). Season with soy sauce, ginger and garlic. Serve the dish with rice or pasta.

**SMOOTHIES**
1. Fruit Salad:
Cut your favorite fruits (such as strawberries, pineapple, kiwi) and mix them in a bowl. Served with whipped cream or yogurt.

2. Chocolate Banana Smoothie: Blend frozen banana, cocoa powder, almond milk, and honey until smooth. Add ice cubes for more thickness.

3. Crispy Apple:
Slice the apple and place it on the baking tray. Mix the flour, oats, brown sugar, and butter in a bowl, then sprinkle it over the apples.
Bake in the oven at 375 degrees Fahrenheit for 30 to 40 minutes, until golden brown.

Conclusion:
With these easy and delicious recipes, you can enjoy healthy, satisfying meals without spending a fortune or spending hours in the kitchen.

Experiment with different ingredients and flavors to create your own signature dish. good food !

# CHAPTER FOUR

# NAVIGATING SOCIAL SITUATIONS AS A RAW FOODIE

As someone who loves to eat raw food, navigating social situations can be challenging.

Whether it's attending a dinner party or eating out with friends, typical social activities often revolve around cooked meals.

Here are some tips to help you handle social situations as a raw foodist:

1. Plan Ahead:

If you know you'll be going to a social event where cooked food will be served, plan ahead by bringing your own fresh food options. This could include a salad, fruit plate, or plate of raw vegetables.

2. Talk to your host:

If you'll be attending a dinner party, talk to your host beforehand about your dietary restrictions. Let them know that you are a fan of fresh food and ask if they can cater for your needs.

3. Be prepared to explain:

When you go out to dinner with friends or family, be prepared to explain your food choices. Some people may not understand why you choose to eat fresh foods, so be prepared to educate them about the benefits.

4. Focus on the Social:
Remember, social events aren't just about food. Focus on the social aspect of the event and enjoy time with friends and family.

5. Take care of yourself:
It is important to take care of yourself when dealing with social situations as a raw person. This may include bringing your own food, setting boundaries, and taking breaks when necessary.

6. Explore new fresh food options: Use social events as an opportunity to explore new fresh food options. Try new recipes and ingredients you may not have tried before.

7. Offer to bring a side dish:
If you're bringing a potluck or barbecue, offer to bring a side dish of raw food that everyone can enjoy. Not only does this ensure you have something to eat, but it also introduces others to the benefits of fresh food.

8. Research restaurants in advance: If you are going to eat out, research restaurants that offer fresh food options in advance. This will save you time and effort searching for something to eat there.

9. Stay hydrated:
Raw foods tend to have a high water content, but it is important to stay hydrated during social events. Bring a reusable water bottle with you and drink water throughout the event.

10. Don't be too hard on yourself: Remember that you can enjoy cooked meals from time to time. Don't be too hard on yourself if you make a mistake at a social event, go back to your raw food lifestyle the next day.
In conclusion, navigating social situations as a raw foodist can be challenging, but with a little planning and communication, you can do it. Remember to focus on the social aspect of the event, take care of yourself, and be prepared to explain your food choices.

# Challenges You May Encounter When Maintaining A Raw Lifestyle in Social Settings Or While Dining Out

1. Limited Options:
When dining out, you may find that the options for fresh food are limited on the menu. This can make it difficult to maintain your raw food lifestyle.

2. Social pressure:
You may experience social pressure from friends or family members who do not understand or support your dietary lifestyle. This can make it difficult to choose your fresh food in a social setting.

3. Attractive smell:
The smell of cooked food can be very attractive, especially if you are hungry or haven't eaten anything in a while. Therefore, it is hard to resist the temptation to enjoy cooked food.

4. Lack of knowledge:
Some restaurants or social events may not have staff who are knowledgeable about fresh food choices, which can make it difficult to make informed choices.

5. Cost:

Raw foods can sometimes be more expensive than cooked foods, which can make it difficult to maintain a raw foods lifestyle when eating out or at social events.

6. Limited Availability:
Depending on where you live, fresh food options may not be available at restaurants or at social events, making it difficult to maintain a fresh, real food lifestyle.

7. Preparation takes time:
Raw dishes can take longer to prepare than cooked dishes, which can be inconvenient when eating out or attending social events.

8. Limited Variety:
Some restaurants offer few fresh food options, which can make it difficult to eat a variety.

9. Misconceptions about raw foods: Some people may have misconceptions about the health benefits of raw foods, which can lead to judgment or criticism from others.

10. Lack of support:
If you don't have a support system or community that understands and supports your raw food lifestyle, it can be difficult for you to stick to it when eating out or attending social events. .

# Practical Advice On How To Handle Situations With Grace And Confidence

Practical advice on how to handle situations safely and with confidence

Life is full of surprises and sometimes we find ourselves in uncomfortable or difficult situations. Whether it's a difficult conversation with a co-worker, a disagreement with a friend, or a stressful event, it's important to know how to handle these situations safely and with confidence.
Some practical tips to help you handle these situations with ease:

1. Stay calm:
The first step to handling any situation with skill and confidence is to remain calm. Breathe deeply and try to stay present. Avoid responding impulsively or emotionally, as this can often lead to actions or words you regret.

2. Active Listening:
When you're having a conversation or disagreeing with someone, make sure you're actively listening to what they're saying.
This means giving them your full attention, asking clarifying questions, and repeating what you've heard to ensure understanding.

3. Choose words carefully:

The words we choose can have a significant impact on the course of a conversation or situation. Pay attention to your accent and language and try to express yourself clearly and respectfully.

4. Finding Common Ground:
In situations of disagreement or conflict, finding common ground can be very helpful. Find areas of agreement or shared value and use them as a starting point for finding a solution or compromise.

5. Empathy:
Empathy is the ability to understand and share the feelings of others. When we practice empathy, we can better relate to others and find solutions that work for everyone involved.

6. Take responsibility:
If you make a mistake or say something hurtful, take responsibility for your actions. Sincerely apologize and take steps to make things right.

7. Take care of yourself:
Taking care of yourself is essential to handling difficult situations safely and confidently. Make sure to prioritize your physical and mental health by getting enough sleep, eating well, and participating in activities that bring you joy.

8. Get help If you're having trouble handling a situation on your own, don't hesitate to ask friends, family, or a professional counselor for help. Having

a support system can make all the difference in dealing with difficult situations.

9. Set boundaries:
It is important to know your limits and to set boundaries in situations where you feel uncomfortable or dangerous. Communicate your boundaries clearly and decisively, and don't be afraid to enforce them if necessary.

10.Be open:
Keeping an open mind can help you approach situations with curiosity and a desire to learn. Avoid making assumptions or jumping to conclusions and be open to new perspectives and ideas.

11. Practice Mindfulness: Mindfulness is the practice of being fully present and aware of the present moment. By practicing mindfulness, you can stay grounded and focused in difficult situations and respond clearly and deliberately.

12. Be positive:
Maintaining a positive attitude can help you approach difficult situations with optimism and flexibility. Focus on the positive aspects of the situation and look for opportunities to grow and learn.

13. Learn from your experience: Every situation can teach us something valuable about ourselves and others. Take time to reflect on your experiences

and use them as opportunities for personal growth and development.

14. Celebrate your successes:
When you've approached a difficult situation with grace and confidence, take time to celebrate your successes.
Recognize your strengths and accomplishments and use them as motivation to take on future challenges.

15. Practice gratitude:
Gratitude is the practice of appreciating the good things in our lives. By focusing on what we are grateful for, we can develop a positive mindset and approach challenging situations with a sense of abundance and possibility.
However, handling situations with skill and confidence takes practice and patience. By staying calm, listening actively, choosing your words carefully, finding common ground, showing empathy, taking responsibility, taking care of yourself, and asking for support when needed, you can handle any situation with ease and confidence.
Remember that every situation is an opportunity to grow and learn.

# CHAPTER FIVE

# Essential Nutrients And Supplements For A Balanced Raw Diet

1. Omega-3 fatty acids:
Found in foods like flaxseeds, chia seeds, and walnuts, these essential fatty acids are important for brain function and can help reduce inflammation.

2. Vitamin B12:
This nutrient is mainly found in animal products, so raw food lovers may need to take supplements to ensure adequate amounts. B12 is important for nerve function and red blood cell production.

3. Iron:
Although iron can be found in plant foods like spinach and lentils, it may not be as easily absorbed as iron found in animal products. Nutritional supplements may be needed to prevent anemia.

4. Vitamin D:
This nutrient is important for bone health and immune function, but getting enough vitamin D from

food alone can be difficult. Dietary supplements or duration of sun exposure may be helpful.

5. Calcium:
Raw fooders may need calcium supplements to ensure they get enough calcium to build strong bones and teeth.

6. Zinc:
This mineral is important for immune function, wound healing, and DNA synthesis. It is found in foods such as pumpkin seeds and cashews, but some foods may require supplementation.

7. Magnesium:
This nutrient is important for muscle and nerve function as well as bone health. It is found in foods such as spinach and almonds, but some foods may require supplementation.

8. Vitamin C:
This antioxidant is important for immune function and collagen production. It is found in foods such as citrus fruits and peppers, but some supplements may be required.

9. Probiotics:
These beneficial bacteria can help improve digestion and boost the immune system. They are found in fermented foods such as sauerkraut and kimchi, or taken as dietary supplements.

10. Fiber:
Raw fooders may need a fiber supplement to ensure adequate fiber intake for digestion and heart health.

11. Selenium:
This mineral is important for thyroid function and immune system health. It is found in foods such as Brazil nuts and mushrooms, but some supplements may be required.

12. Vitamin K:
This nutrient is important for blood clotting and bone health. It is found in green leafy vegetables such as kale and spinach, but some may require supplementation.

13. Coenzyme Q10:
This antioxidant is important for energy production and heart health. It can be found in foods such as fatty fish and offal, but some foods may require supplementation.

14. Lycopene:
This antioxidant is important for heart health and may help reduce the risk of some types of cancer. It can be found in foods like tomatoes and watermelon, or taken as a supplement.

15. Choline:

This nutrient is important for brain function and liver health. It can be found in foods such as eggs and liver, but some foods may require supplementation.

16. Iodine:
This mineral is important for thyroid function and can be found in seaweed and iodized salt, but for some people, supplementation may be necessary.

17. Vitamin E:
This antioxidant is important for healthy skin and immune function. It is found in foods such as almonds and sunflower seeds, but some supplements may be required.

18. Chromium:
This mineral is important for regulating blood sugar and can be found in foods like broccoli and barley, but for some people, supplementation may be necessary.

19. Manganese:
This mineral is important for bone health and wound healing. It is found in foods such as whole grains and nuts, but some types may need supplementation.

20. Phosphorus:
This mineral is important for bone health and energy production. It can be found in foods such as salmon and lentils, but some foods may require supplementation.

21. Potassium:
This mineral is important for heart health and muscle function. It is found in foods such as bananas and sweet potatoes, but some foods may require supplementation.

22. Vitamin A:
This nutrient is important for vision and immune function. It can be found in foods such as carrots and sweet potatoes, but some foods may require supplementation.

23. Vitamin B6:
This nutrient is important for brain function and can be found in foods such as chickpeas and bananas, but additional supplementation may be required some.

24. Vitamin B9 (folic acid):
This nutrient is important for fetal development and can be found in foods such as green vegetables and legumes, but some types may require supplementation.

25. Vitamin B1 (thiamine): This nutrient is important for energy production and can be found in foods such as whole grains and pork, but some types may require supplementation.

26. Vitamin B2 (riboflavin):

This nutrient is important for energy production and can be found in foods such as dairy products and green vegetables, but some types may require supplementation.

27. Vitamin B3 (Niacin):
This nutrient is important for energy production and can be found in foods such as meat and legumes, but for some people, supplementation may be necessary.

28. Vitamin B5 (pantothenic acid): This nutrient is important for energy production and can be found in foods like avocados and mushrooms, but some types may require supplementation.

29. Vitamin H (Biotin):
This nutrient is important for healthy hair and nails and can be found in foods like eggs and nuts, but some may require supplementation.

30. Vitamin E (inositol):
This nutrient is important for nerve function and can be found in foods such as citrus fruits and beans, but some types may require supplementation.

31. Vitamin P (bioflavonoids):
This antioxidant is important for immune function and can be found in foods such as berries and citrus fruits, but some may require supplementation.

32. Vitamin T (rutin):
This antioxidant is important for healthy blood vessels and can be found in foods like buckwheat and citrus fruits, but some people may need it.

33. Vitamin U (S-methylmethionine): This nutrient is important for a healthy stomach and can be found in foods like cabbage and beets, but some types may require supplementation.

34. Silica:
This mineral is important for healthy bones and connective tissues and can be found in foods such as oats and cucumbers, but some types may require supplementation.

35. Boron:
This mineral is important for bone health and can be found in foods such as almonds and avocados, but some may require supplementation.

36. Vanadium:
This mineral is important for regulating blood sugar and can be found In foods such as mushrooms and shellfish, but for some people, supplementation may be necessary.

37. Copper:
This mineral is important for nerve function and can be found in foods like liver and shellfish, but for some people, supplementation may be necessary.

38. Molybdenum:
This mineral is important for enzyme function and can be found in foods such as lentils and spinach, but some types may need supplementation.

39. Nickel:
This mineral is important for enzyme function and can be found in foods such as nuts and legumes, but some types may require supplementation.

40. Tin:
This mineral is important for immune function and can be found in foods such as canned tomatoes and seafood, but some types may require supplementation.

41. Lutein:
This antioxidant is important for eye health and can be found in foods like spinach and kale, but some foods may require supplementation.

42. Zeaxanthin:
This antioxidant is important for eye health and can be found in foods like corn and peppers, but some supplements may be needed.

43. Omega-6 fatty acids:
Found in foods like nuts, these essential fatty acids are important for brain function and can help reduce inflammation, but too much can be harmful.

A balanced omega-3 and omega-6 supplement is recommended.

44. Glucosamine:
This nutrient is important for joint health and can be found in oysters and bone broth, but some people may need supplements.

45. Chondroitin:
This nutrient is important for joint health and can be found in animal cartilage, but for some people, supplementation may be necessary.

46. MSM (methylsulfonylmethane): This nutrient is important for joint health and can be found in foods like broccoli and garlic, but for some people, supplementation may be necessary.

47. Ashwagandha:
This herb is known for its anti-stress properties and can be taken as a dietary supplement.

48. Rhodiola:
This herb is known for its stimulant properties and can be taken as a nutritional supplement.

49. Ginkgo biloba:
This herb is known for its memory-enhancing properties and can be taken as a dietary supplement.

50. Ginseng:

This herb is known for its adaptogenic properties and can help improve energy, reduce stress and boost the immune system. It can be taken as a supplement.

## Recommendations on sources of essential vitamins, minerals and other vital Nutrients

1. Fruits and vegetables: Include a variety of colorful fruits and vegetables in your diet to ensure you are getting a variety of essential vitamins, minerals and nutrients.

2.Whole grains: Choose whole grain products like brown rice, whole grain bread and oatmeal to get essential nutrients like B vitamins, iron and fiber.

3. Lean meat and fish: Include lean cuts of meat such as chicken or turkey and fatty fish such as salmon or sardines for high-quality protein, omega-3 fatty acids and various minerals.

4. Dairy Products: Eat dairy products such as milk, yogurt, and cheese to get calcium, vitamin D, and other nutrients needed for bone health.

5. Legumes: Include legumes and beans such as lentils, chickpeas, and kidney beans in your diet to get vegetable protein, fiber, iron, and vitamins.

6. Nuts: Snack on a variety of nuts such as almonds, walnuts, chia seeds, and flaxseeds to get healthy fats, protein, and essential vitamins and minerals.

7. Eggs: Include eggs in your diet as they are full of high-quality protein and vitamins and minerals like choline, zinc and vitamin B12.

8. Healthy fats: Incorporate healthy fats from sources such as avocados, olive oil, and nuts into your diet to get important vitamins (such as vitamin E) and essential fatty acids.

9. Fortified foods: Consider fortified foods such as fortified cereals, breads and plant-based milk alternatives to make sure you get enough essential nutrients such as calcium, iron and vitamin D.

10. Seafood: Eat seafood such as shrimp, mussels, and oysters to get essential nutrients like iodine, selenium, and omega-3 fatty acids.

11. Dark leafy vegetables: Eat dark leafy vegetables such as spinach, kale, and Swiss chard because they are rich in vitamins A, C, K, and various minerals.

12. Citrus: Enjoy citrus fruits such as oranges, grapefruits, and lemons because they contain vitamin C, folic acid, and potassium.

13. Cruciferous vegetables: Incorporate cruciferous vegetables like broccoli, Brussels sprouts, and cauliflower into your diet for a variety of vitamins, minerals, and antioxidants.

14. Berries: Snack on berries like strawberries, raspberries, and blueberries to get antioxidants, vitamins, and fiber.

15. Bell peppers: Incorporate different colored bell peppers into your meals to get essential vitamins A, C, and E, as well as antioxidants.

16. Sweet Potatoes: Enjoy sweet potatoes as they are a good source of vitamin A, fiber and other essential nutrients.

17. Mushrooms: Include a variety of mushrooms in your diet to get B vitamins, selenium, and other important nutrients.

18. Herbs and Spices: Use a variety of herbs and spices such as turmeric, cinnamon, and oregano in your cooking to enhance flavor and bring in a variety of beneficial compounds.

19. Fermented foods: Include fermented foods like yogurt, kefir, sauerkraut, and kimchi to boost gut health and get beneficial probiotics.

20. Seaweed: Add seaweed to your diet to get iodine, iron and other essential minerals.

21. Quinoa: Replace your regular grains with quinoa for a complete source of protein, fiber, and various vitamins and minerals.

22. Lentils: Enjoy lentils as they are full of fiber, protein, iron and other important nutrients.

23. Chia seeds: Add chia seeds to your meals or drinks to get omega-3 fatty acids, fiber and important minerals like calcium and magnesium.

24. Flaxseed: Sprinkle ground flaxseed into meals or stir it into baked goods for omega-3 fatty acids and fiber.

25. Hemp seeds: Include hemp seeds in your diet to get plant-based protein, omega-3 fatty acids, and essential minerals like magnesium and zinc.

26. Pumpkin Seeds: Use pumpkin seeds to get loads of nutrients like magnesium, zinc, iron, and antioxidants.

27. Sunflower seeds: Enjoy sunflower seeds as a snack for vitamin E, selenium and essential minerals.

28. Oysters: Add oysters to your diet to provide a rich source of zinc, iron, vitamin B12 and omega-3 fatty acids.

29. Brazil nuts: Snack on Brazil nuts to get more selenium, a mineral important for thyroid function and antioxidant protection.

30. Almonds: Enjoy almonds as a snack or include them in your meals to get healthy fats, vitamin E and important minerals.

31. Nuts: Snack on nuts to get omega-3 fatty acids, antioxidants and various beneficial compounds.

32. Cashews: Include cashews in your diet to get healthy fats, minerals like magnesium and zinc, and important vitamins.

# CHAPTER SIX

# CONCLUSION

# SUSTAINING MOTIVATION AND OVERCOMING COMMON OBSTACLES

Motivation drives our actions and plays an important role in achieving our goals.

However, staying motivated can be challenging as we often encounter obstacles that stand in the way of our progress.

In this book, we'll explore effective strategies for staying motivated and overcoming common obstacles along the way.

Set clear and realistic goals:

To stay motivated, it is essential to set clear, specific, and achievable goals. Break larger goals into smaller, more manageable tasks to maintain a sense of progress and achievement.

Make sure your goals align with your values and aspirations, giving them personal meaning.

2.Find the "why":

Determining the reasons behind achieving the goal can be a powerful motivator. Think about the purpose and meaning of your goal. Understanding the "why" of your actions can help you stay focused and engaged, even in the face of obstacles.

3. Maintain a positive mindset:

A positive mindset is crucial to staying motivated. Cultivate confidence and optimism by focusing on your strengths and past successes.

Surround yourself with positive influences and get inspired by others facing similar challenges. Accept failure as a learning experience and an opportunity for growth.

4. Break the task into manageable steps:

Feeling overwhelmed by the importance of a goal can take a toll on motivation. Break your tasks down into smaller, more manageable steps.

This approach allows you to focus on one task at a time, reducing stress and increasing your chances of success. Celebrate every achievement to stay motivated.

5. Web development support:

Building a support network of like-minded people can provide encouragement, empowerment, and motivation.

Share your goals and progress with trusted friends, family, or mentors who can provide you with constructive support and feedback. Participating in peer groups or online communities related to your goals can also provide valuable insight and motivation.

6. Create a routine:

Establishing a consistent routine can help stay motivated by eliminating decision fatigue and increasing productivity.
Set a specific time each day or week to achieve your goal. By prioritizing goals in your schedule, you'll be more likely to stay motivated and cut through distractions.

7. Be flexible and adaptable:
Obstacles and failures are inevitable in any journey. Instead of getting discouraged, see them as opportunities to learn and grow. Maintain a flexible mindset and be willing to adapt your approach to challenges.
Accept that setbacks are temporary and part of the process of achieving success.

## Common Hurdles That Individuals may face while pursuing a raw food lifestyle

1 Lack of knowledge about raw food preparation techniques, difficulties in finding new and membership products throughout the year
2 Temptation to return to unhealthy eating habits
3 Social and important social pressure from friends and family
4 Options for the process of recovery or participating in social events.
5 Cooked or manufactured food desire
6 Preparing and planning meals over time
7 Votes about buying high -quality ingredients
8 Deficiency or imbalance in foodstuffs
9 Difficulties in the transition period
10 Emotional relationship with some of the bent foods on supporting the local community or colleagues
11 Difficulty finding a raw restaurant or cafe
12 Reactions or negative assessment of others about many recipes and raw foods
13 Inability to maintain a balanced raw diet while traveling
14 Restricted access to fresh food components at reasonable prices 15 bored with frequent raw dishes
16 Need an additional additional diet
17 lack of energy or fatigue in the initial steps
18 unrealistic expectation to improve health immediately
19 Fear of missing cultural or traditional food

20 Difficult in obtaining raw food ingredients in rural areas

21 It is restricted or not in a mixer or a food robot

22 It is difficult to find enough protein sources in the raw diet

23 lack of motivation or discipline to comply with the diet

24 lack of knowledge about the appropriate mix of food on the raw diet

25 symptoms of pulling food

26 Fear of judgment or the absurdity of others

27 The overwhelming desire for an emotional or stressful position

28 Killer with unhealthy food temptations at work

29 Do not meet the fear of food needs, especially for children or athletes

29 Time restrictions due to work or other obligations

30 Difficulty in finding raw food ingredients with a limited budget

31 Far to miss your favorite cooking dishes

32 Uncomfortable or swelling in the process of consuming a large amount of raw foods

33 Feeling of isolation or difference between others who do not follow the raw diet

34 Decreased dining skills to create delicious raw dishes

35 Lack of knowledge about the appropriate food storage techniques and storage

36 The ability to eat naturally due to the limited raw food options

# Strategies For Staying Motivated And Overcoming These Obstacles To Maintain Long Term Success

Set clear, specific, achievable goals: 1. Clearly define what you want to achieve and engage in smaller, manageable tasks.

2. Create a vision board:
Visualize your goals by creating a vision board that includes images and phrases that inspire and motivate you.

3. Develop a positive mindset: Develop a positive attitude towards challenges and failures, and believe in your ability to overcome them.

4. Surround yourself with positive influences:
Surround yourself with people who support and encourage your goals, Avoid negative or toxic people who bring you down.

5. Celebrate small victories: Acknowledge and celebrate small steps along the way to keep your motivation high.

6. Learn from failures:
Instead of wallowing in failures, see them as learning opportunities. Analyze what went wrong and use that knowledge to improve.

7. Take care of yourself:
Take care of your physical, mental and emotional health. Get enough sleep, exercise regularly, eat nutritious foods, and practice relaxation techniques.

8. Break tasks into smaller steps: Break important tasks into smaller, more manageable steps. It will make the journey less painful and give a sense of progress.

9. Create a habit:
Create a daily routine that includes time set aside for achieving your goals. Consistency creates motivation and success.

10. Reward yourself:
Set rewards for reaching milestones to maintain high levels of motivation.

11. Find your "why": Identify the deeper reasons and motivations behind your goals. Understanding your "why" will give you a solid foundation to stay motivated.

12. Keep Learning:
Continuously strive to develop knowledge and skills relevant to your goals. Learning new things keeps your mind busy and energizes your motivation.

13. Seek Support:

Connect with mentors, coaches, or like-minded people who can offer advice, support, and encouragement.

14.Gratitude:
Focus on what you have achieved and be grateful for the progress you have made. Gratitude promotes a positive mental state and motivation.

15. Visualize Success:
Visualize yourself achieving your goals and experiencing the success you desire. Use visualization techniques to boost your motivation.

16. Stay organized:
Use tools like calendars, to-do lists, and planners to stay organized and on track with your tasks and goals.

17. Accept Failure as part of the journey. Understand that failure is a natural part of the success process. Accept it, learn from it, and keep moving forward.